Food Addiction

The What, Why, & Solutions for Emotional Eating

by Cathy Wilson
Copyright © 2014

Income Disclaimer

This book contains business strategies, marketing methods and other business advice that, regardless of my own results and experience, may not produce the same results (or any results) for you. I make absolutely no guarantee, expressed or implied, that by following the advice below you will make any money or improve current profits, as there are several factors and variables that come into play regarding any given business.

Primarily, results will depend on the nature of the product or business model, the conditions of the marketplace, the experience of the individual, and situations and elements that are beyond your control.

As with any business endeavor, you assume all risk related to investment and money based on your own discretion and at your own potential expense.

Liability Disclaimer

By reading this book, you assume all risks associated with using the advice given below, with a full understanding that you, solely, are responsible for anything that may occur as a result of putting this information into action in any way, and regardless of your interpretation of the advice.

You further agree that our company cannot be held responsible in any way for the success or failure of your business as a result of the information presented in this book. It is your responsibility to conduct your own due diligence regarding the safe and successful operation of your business if you intend to apply any of our information in any way to your business operations.

Terms of Use

You are given a non-transferable, "personal use" license to this book. You cannot distribute it or share it with other individuals.

Also, there are no resale rights or private label rights granted when purchasing this book. In other words, it's for your own personal use only.

Food Addiction

The What, Why, & Solutions for Emotional Eating

by Cathy Wilson

Table of Contents

Introduction

Do you find your mind wandering to thoughts of that lusciously sweet bowl of chocolate covered strawberries you indulge in EVERY Saturday night? It's the one that seems to be increasing steadily with each passing week?

Or how about planning your day so that you have ample time, even if caught in traffic, to get your 6 pack of beer religiously every weekday on your way home?

Food addiction is a serious issue that often creeps up when least expected, by the time we recognize ourselves craving more and more of a particular unhealthy food.

The handcuffs are already on and we're on route to the tank whether we want to or not. At this point, we're passed the point of just habit and have totally lost control. When you don't control a particular eating habit or are negatively affected when you don't happen to get your "fix," this is a food addiction. It's common in our society today and extremely harmful. But, until you actually learn how to set your pride aside and overtly admit and recognize you are suffering, the cycle of destruction will continue.

Using my 20 plus years of health and wellness experience, my dietician studies, research and first hand personal experiences, I will introduce to you food addiction, factors in food addiction and most importantly solutions to help you take control of your eating and life. YOU deserve to be happy and in order to do this you've got to step up to the plate and regain control of what you eat, when and how much.

Is this going to be easy?

Absolutely not. Likely one of the hardest things in life you've had to do.

Can *you do it?*
That's affirmative. I know and you know you can do it and I'm going to give you the tools showing you how. What you need to do is take positive action to slowly but surely remove your negativity associated with food, re-learning the joy of what controlled healthy food choices does for your mind, body and soul.

Take from this book, the factors that make sense to you. Apply them considering your tolerances and preferences to create a personal plan of action geared specially for you. What works for hunky Fed Ex driver Hank and sweet little Cindy Lou-Who down the street isn't going to work for you.

Expect to fall a few times. Just commit to getting right back up and onward you go.
Commit your mind strong to not letting ANYTHING and I mean ANYTHING get in your way. You'll know why when you reach the finish line.

Mind over matter folks. This book will give you ample fire power but it's up to you to open your mind and grow the balls to pull the trigger. And don't pretend you don't know exactly what I mean!

What is Food Addiction?

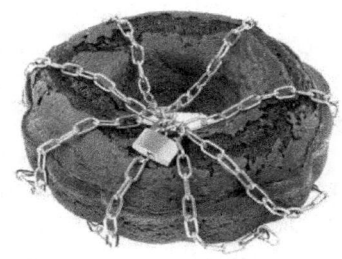

Food addiction is anything but simple, affecting you negatively on so many life levels. Your social, mental, physical and emotional character is extremely susceptible to influence with food addiction. First, let's look at what addiction is…

Addiction is – the inability to have conscious control of your eating. That's the basic skin and bones of it, having an addiction suggest you lack control in what you are using, taking or doing to a point that's harmful. It can refer to a substance dependency, like drugs, or a behavioral addiction, like online gambling.

Society naturally associates addiction with physical substances and for our purpose we are going with food addiction, although as you can see addiction is diverse, wide and very deep.

Being addicted is a self-created dependency, a mechanism is which your cope in everyday life.

Food Addiction is – simple the inability to control eating, whether it's a specific type of food or quantity doesn't matter. The fact that you have taught yourself to depend on food adds up to food addiction.

It's a difficult scenario because as humans we need food to survive. It's not like a substance abuse addiction where you have the opportunity for TOTAL avoidance to remove the issue of temptation and increase the odds of success.

With an addiction to food you are constantly reminded of it because you are dependent on the base substance you're abusing, just in different parameters of course. If you are addicted to sweets you physically need them for survival, although sometimes you may feel this way. BUT, when you are eating your usual healthy dinner you're reminded of how much you are craving your sweets and this makes it more difficult to treat, get rid of or control your food craving. Sort of like getting dumped unexpectedly and having to see the "dumpee" every day, only to remind you of what could have been. Making it harder to get over the sap and get on with life. Does that make sense?

A few other pointers on food addiction to put into your brain for future reference:

Food addiction is maladaptive. What the beep does that mean? Well that regardless of the fact people often over-eat to feel better, mentally speaking. This destructive act often leaves them feeling worse off, triggering symptoms of ugliness, guilt, embarrassment and less validity in general.

FACT – An addiction to food can eventually kill you. Causing interference with the healthy running of your in-

ternal circuits, obesity, mental stresses and all sorts of
other issues that won't make you smile, a good cry would
be more appropriate.

*Food addiction is CONSTANTLY there, always persis-
tent.* This, in itself, is very difficult to deal with. Tough to
change something or forget about it what it's always in
your face, agreed? Nobody is perfect and particularly
around the holidays we all overeat some. No worries
there because that's where it stops. Someone with a food
addiction makes habit of overeating and often uses it as
a mechanism to cope with stress. In time, this develops
into a frequent daily need and when it doesn't happen,
anxiousness kicks in.

**There's a pattern of destruction often hidden for fear
of negative consequence, disappointment or disap-
proval of others. As humans, we have learned to rely
heavily on the opinions of others and often this
sways our actions, thinking one thing and doing another.**

Are Habit and Addiction the Same?
Technically no, but they're interconnected.
HABIT is what you do consciously by choice. There is no
loss of control here or psychological issue. You can make
a habit of going to the gym each morning to blast your
body into shape for sexy summertime. Then when you
get tired of dragging your butt out of bed so early in the
morning to fulfill this habit, you can just stop. Sure there's
a consequence. In this case, it's getting fat. But the key is
this is CONTROLLABLE. If you want to restart your habit
you can.

ADDICTION, as we've discussed, doesn't have that "controlled" component. The physical and psychological take
over and transform your actions or habit into a need or

absolute. An addiction can't simply be turned on and off like a habit. It's much more complex.

Key Factor in Addiction – Over time, you will need more and more as your tolerance level will become conditioned. It's accommodating and getting used to a particular substance, action or thought process, forcing you to need MORE physically and psychologically, acting as a game of dominos, driving you become MORE addicted, connected on a deeper level. Suffice to say, the longer this process continues, the deep the hole you'll have to dig yourself out of.

EXAMPLE – Honestly, drugs or alcohol addiction are the first to come to mind here, but we're going to use food. Let's say you make a habit of eating high sugar sweets at the end of the day, when you finally get a minute to sit down on the couch and watch a couple hours of television. You may begin having just a small bowl of chips, a few smarties and maybe a glass of soda.

Initially, this satiated your learned after dinner sugar craving and your psychological need to feel "rewarded" for a hard day's work. It's not healthy, but often a reality for many.

SMARTER CHOICE! A better choice would be to go to the gym for an hour and "reward" yourself with a scrumptious fruit smoothie and maybe a bowl of pretzels while watching an hour of television.

After a few weeks of your high-sugar, low nutrition constant sugar surge after dinner, something internally triggers you to slowly, but surely increase the amount you're eating. Your body and mind both mentally and physically quickly learn your temporary "feel good feeling" is stronger with more sweets. Of course you're not thinking straight, driven by the need for increased glucose levels after dinner and you just keep proper the amount of time spent eating these foods and the amounts. Eventually, your mind will take control more and you will find yourself planning and thinking about your evening eating ritual, making plans to ensure you get your "addiction" fulfilled. Nothing else matters.

After the fact chances are you're going to come down hard and feel bad or guilty about your deep dark dirty little secret. But you will brush these thoughts off and lie to yourself that you don't have an addiction and that you will cut back "next time."
Sound familiar?

I bet my right arm and leg if I have to that you know exactly what I'm talking about. I know I do.
It's only when you know you've had enough and you seriously want to change, wWhen you TELL others about it and TALK about it openly you're ready to start making the changes to manage your food addiction. It's a choice, YOUR choice.

VERY CRITICAL NOTE! Please know that having an addiction, food or otherwise is NOT something to be ashamed or embarrassed about. Admitting this is something wonderful, courageous and meaningful because every single person on the face of the earth has hidden secrets they aren't strong enough to battle. It's not a judgment, just a reality.

By taking action to battle your demons you are demonstrating to the rest of us just how awesome you are. That's what I believe for what it's worth!

My Thoughts…

Understanding the basic differences between habit, addiction and food addiction is imperative in the game of life. The more knowledge you have and better yet pull from your unconscious to your conscious thoughts and apply, the better.

These introductory concepts are exactly what you need to get all fired up to move onto the next chapter. You've got to be wondering by now what triggers food addiction right?

Causal Factors

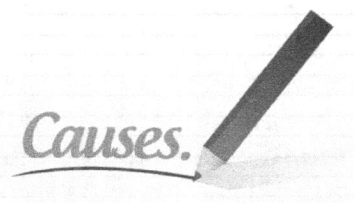

If foods you know are unhealthy for you, they are constantly calling your name. If you are finding it harder and harder to say no to that second bag of potato chips or find yourself dipping into yet another bag of your favorite cookies when you're light-years passed full, then you've likely got a food addiction, depending on how long you've been experiencing these symptoms and your actions when they arise.

FACT- We KNOW healthy eating is important in overall good health and wellness. Moderation is key and your body is NOT programmed to need any sort of sweet treats to optimize your health.

This means nutritionally you don't need chips, pastries, butter, cookies, candy bars, soda and so forth. The intrinsic of your body can do fine without them.

What happens is your mind takes control here. Slowly, but surely you create the psychological need for this overeating and use it as an escape. Maybe, over time you use overeating to drown your sorrows when dumped, or perhaps whenever you have a "bad" day you use the sugar rush you receive to make yourself feel better. At least that's what you tell yourself and that's exactly what happens temporarily, which is all the "proof" you need to keep on trucking.

It doesn't help that these unhealthy fast-foods and sugary sweets are within arm's reach always. It's not like way back in "Little House on the Prairie" days when you had to walk five miles into town if you needed to buy some extra bread. This forced interference and made you think long and hard if you REALLY needed that bread or if you could just make due waiting for another half day for "ma" to get hers baked.

Times have changed and we live in a VERY dangerous environment food-wise. You don't even have to think about eating a chocolate bar, the consequences and whether or not you're really hungry for it or not. Because it's out of the wrapper and down the hatch before you take your next breath. You don't even give your mind enough time to talk yourself into eating a stalk of celery or banana with peanut butter instead.

I understand I'm rambling a little, but it is so critical to recognize how easy it is to slip and fall here, a far harder task to stay on track to making the right food choices, understanding moderation and steering yourself clear of falling into the nastily deep trap of food addiction.

To add to your information overload, food expert and former FDA Commissioner Dr. David Kessler believes strongly there are similarities between sugary foods and drug addiction. Makes sense, but just complicates things. He talks often about "hyperpalatable foods." These are foods loaded with fats and sugars that reward us in giving us the internal need to want more, eating high sugar foods naturally stimulates endorphin release. It's similar to that "feel good feeling" you get when exercising. Without knowing or even recognizing initially, this sugary food eating becomes habit and it's that simulated endorphin release that solidifies the deal, leaving you wanting, needing and craving more.

Causes of Food Addiction
Experts agree there isn't one causal factor for food addiction. It's a multifactorial issue that needs all areas addressed.
BIOLOGICAL
SOCIAL
PSYCHOLOGICAL
All play a role in becoming addicted to food.
The Biological…
*hormonal imbalance
*structural brain abnormalities
*genetics
*consequences of taking certain powerful drugs

Researchers agree there are some factors in food addiction you don't have control of that naturally increase your risk of developing food addictive habits under particular circumstance. This cannot be used as an excuse though because even if food addictive tendencies run in the family and your brain may be a little more wired to wanting sugar, this doesn't mean you have to eat more sugary foods. It means you need to be a little stronger in the sugar department and take more pro-active action in prevention.

STEER CLEAR OF THE MIDDLE ISLES IN THE GROCERY STORY BECAUSE THAT'S WHERE ALL THE SUGAR IS STORED!
The Social…
*abnormal family function
*societal pressures, real or unreal

19

*family and friend pressures
*abuse during childhood, sexually or verbally
*stress in general
*isolation
*little to no social support
*no friends
*media

This one is tough because if you happen to be hanging out with a bunch of sugar junkies for example, saying no means you aren't "conforming" socially, an intrinsic need we require and search for as human beings. This is where you need to take a stand to just stay away from these external pressures so that you aren't going to develop a NEED for unhealthy eating. Again, it's a choice. Tough or not, you have to make it.

VIP!!!! I think it's important to note how dangerous the media can be when it comes to food addiction and young girls in particular. We live in a society driven by external social factors. Slim and trim is associated with sexy and sexy gets you in the door to being wanted and accepted. Nobody wants to be ugly or normal. Everyone wants to be skinny, sexy, popular, and drop dead gorgeous.

Young girls put such a high value on being "the one" guys are talking about that they will do whatever it takes to fit the profile. Often abusing food is one avenue. Extremes are developed and when a young girl feels they don't fit the bill they quite easily throw in the towel and flip to the other extreme of existence. They will let themselves go, drowning themselves in unhealthy foods.

Their mindset?

Well distorted logic tells them they might as well reward themselves with sinful sugars because they are NEVER going to be thin and beautiful. Temporarily convincing themselves that a food addiction of sugar really does make them happy. Thus begins the cycle of self-destruction. In time, when fat, tired and developing serious health issues, the truth emerges, realizing this doesn't make them happy and now they are in so deep literally they're unsure what to do, forcing extreme measures to be taken regardless.

I know this because I lived it.
We really don't realize how influential young girls and guys for that matter, really are. Even the confident ones are just as susceptible as anyone else to fall prey to the realities of our world, one of which is the increasingly dangerous world of food addiction. Think about that the next time to comment to anyone about their appearance.

The Psychological...
*verbal or sexual abuse
*trauma survivor
*deeply hidden secrets unbearable
*low self-confidence
*naturally naïve
*depressed or other mental conditions

Here food often ends up being used as a coping mechanism for a hidden weakness. Rather than face life challenges some choose to ignore or run from them and often placing food in the limelight for "dealing" with this stress is what people choose.

Bottom line is that food addiction is a very serious mental health issue that needs to be addressed. The consequences will continue to escalate and are serious from the start, a moment in time where you need to just take action. Don't stop and think about things because if you continue to do so you are just increasing the chances you'll just curdle and continue your destructive food addiction ways. You know it, I know it, and now it's time for you to act on this. Only YOU can make the changes necessary.

My Thoughts…
Understanding some of the triggers or causes that often create poor eating habits that can eventually turn into addictive eating is critical. You need to know the causes of your actions in order to understand better which weapon you need to make in preparation for battle.
Grab your weapon and prepare for battle.

Signals of it

We're going deep and here with the signs and symptoms of food addiction, using my personal experience combined with all the research and medical based knowledge I've amassed over the years. So much, it truly is scary! It's worth it though so that I can deliver to you even just one pointer that will help you improve your quality of life. It's time for you to get a little overwhelmed and probably experience a little familiar recognition.

Signals of Food Addiction

*Your mind wanders to unhealthy foods routinely
*Looking forward to unhealthy eating sessions
*Planning your day around unhealthy eating
*Getting pissy if you happen to miss your "fix" on occasion
*Finding your energy levels on a roller coaster ride
*Changing your normal plans to get a specific food regularly
*Choosing eating sessions over work or social engagements
*Ignoring hunger cues you are full to have more and more of a certain food

*Tummy troubles
*Experiencing crazy nuts mood swings
*Trouble getting to sleep
*Decreased quality of sleep
*Really tough to get out bed in the morning
*Hard to focus and concentrate
*Less patience
*Eating so much you feel like barfing
*Overspending on particularly fatty foods whether you can afford it or not
*Radical thinking, suicidal thoughts
*Your food thoughts seem to be taking over your life
Any of these sound familiar?

RECOGNITION is the first step of the solution. You need to first come to terms with the fact you might very well have a food addiction that needs to be taken care of. It's all about opening your mind, setting your ego aside and gaining the courage you need to face this issue. Sure you can hide forever, but eventually your food addiction will kill you. Worst case scenario, it will jeopardize your good health to the extreme.

After all is said and done, leaving you WISHING you had taken action years sooner. Now is the time for you to make a change for the better in YOUR life. As always, it's up to you to take that first most difficult step.

My Thoughts…
Understanding, opening your thoughts to recognizing and accepting you have signs or symptoms associated with a food addiction is step one. This needs to happen if you are going to move forward positively in creating YOUR plan to manage and beat your food addiction. It's something you will have to choose to change because one thing for certain is it's not going to just magically disappear. Wishful thinking though…

24

The Extremes – Bulimia and Anorexia Nervosa Explained

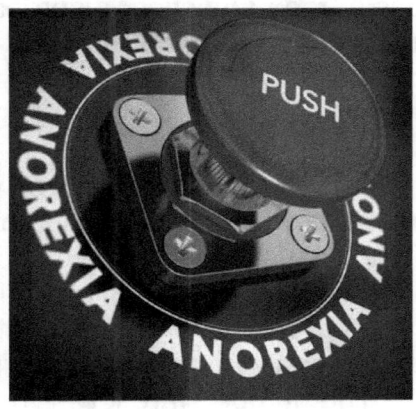

Extreme in anything is NOT a good thing. Being too nice will set you up to be taken advantage of. Too smart will increase pressures always "expecting" you to have the answers. Going to the gym too much will cause overtraining which can be just as damaging as not working out at all.

When it comes to extremes in eating there are two common eating disorders that pop to mind. Chances are you've at least heard of both. I'm going to deepen your knowledge a little and hopefully project some positive light you can use to help yourself get healthier in life. Often being aware of your enemies gives you the one up! I don't want to get in too deep here as this book is geared to give you the beginner's knowledge in food addiction. However, I do feel strongly it's important for you and the rest of the world to take a few minutes to better understand these eating disorders that affect so many more people you love and care about than you think.

Bulimia

Bulimia isn't as popular as anorexia, but it's definitely recognizable in society today. This detrimental psychological disease is a "food addiction" disorder where you overeat regularly and then try and make up for it by exercising to the extreme, abusing laxatives or making yourself throw up.

It's where you experience a loss of control with food and can't help yourself from sometimes eating over 3,400 calories in a sitting. Usually fatty, high-calorie foods are the crutch and the guilt afterwards is most unbearable. The *National Health Services Board* states that up to 8% of the female population will suffer from bulimia at some point in their life. The numbers are lower for men, but still relevant.

Why?
As we've already covered above, bulimia is caused mainly by genetics, abuse, trauma, societal pressures and other mental health issues.

Signs and Symptoms
*GUILT
*OVEREATING
*PURGING
These are the three main signals you're suffering from bulimia.

The guilt arises because you do recognize you've lost control. Self-esteem takes a beating and you just "feel" fat whether you are or aren't. It's a destructive cycle leaving you feeling helpless, afraid, and alone. Even when

26

you set your mind to stop it, you always end up falling back into your destructive eating ways.

The overeating is mainstay. No matter what you tell yourself you always seem to end up in your favorite chair eating crazy amounts of high-fat foods. Doesn't matter that you know how unhealthy this is. Your head tells you this is what you need to do in order to feel "better," so that's exactly what you do.

It's only termed overeating or binge eating when you do it regularly. You probably plan these episodes and often look forward to them, a signal you do have a very real issue to deal with.

Purging is your reaction to loss of self-control. This is where you feel fat, ugly and just plain awful. The temporary solution is to get rid of this feeling as quickly as possible, taking extreme measures in triggering vomiting, abusing laxatives or hitting the gym for hours on end to try and burn off all that extra fat and calories.

A few other indicators associated with people suffering from bulimia are...
-Constant flips and dips in body weight
-Setting extra money aside for food
-Secrecy
-Abnormal exercise patterns
-Anxiousness and depression
-Extreme mood swings
-Puffy face
-Dental issues
-Unhappy body image
-Red eyes
-Whacky periods (girls)
-Continuous throat/nose issues

Keep in mind that just because you recognize some of these symptoms in yourself or a loved one doesn't cement the fact they have developed bulimia. These are just indicators suggesting they might.

Consequences
Complications can arise mild to extreme when suffering from bulimia, including
*poor mineral absorption
*rotten teeth
*stomach problems
*fat fingers because of laxative abuse
*unhealthy skin and hair
*self-induced chemical imbalance triggering extreme tiredness, convulsions, kidney and heart damage
*throat swelling
*chronic constipation
*dehydration
*drug abuse
*loss or irregular monthly period
*Heightened mental conditions like depression, anxiety and phobias

Solutions/Treatment
Experts in the medical profession offer a variety of treatment options for bulimia. Ultimately the most successful combination includes:
-Family counselling
-Psychotherapy
-Medication
-Healthy eating counselling
Critical here, is ensuring the patient understands there is a mental component that needs professional guidance and support. This isn't something that someone can typically manage and step past on their own, at least not indefinitely.

Dips, dives, twists and turns in life often trigger relapses even when in treatment. So you can imagine the scenario flying solo with no support.

The National Health Services supports the belief the first step that MUST happen is realizing you're suffering from a sickness/disease/illness. And knowing that if you truly want to take action and get better this is going to involve a gynormous lifestyle change, creation of new healthy habits and a persistence to commit to this forever.

"Food," in the larger sense is something you have to face each day, a reminder of your particular food addiction continuously. Mentally you need to build your mind strong enough to get passed your internal desires to get your "food fix" and continuously focus on establishing and practicing health eating. Definitely doable, but not easy.

Strategy Treatment
Needs to include…
-You, the patient
-Partner and/or immediate family
-Medical practitioner
-Psychologist or mental healthcare provider
-Nutritionist or eating specialist expert in eating disorders

Treatment Option One - Psychotherapy
The first move is to help establish a positive and healthy relationship with food. A psychologist will help you understand how you feel about food and eating and transform these thoughts positively, ensuring you understand and realize you have an eating disorder and with your approval work at getting your thoughts healthy with regards to food, body weight and everything food related – feelings, behaviors and actions.
In psychotherapy, treatment focuses on thoughts and behavior, cognitive and behavioral therapy respectively.

Over time, realistic and healthy thoughts, feelings and behaviors are developed towards eating and nutrition in general, along with coping mechanism to handle every-day stresses that might very well cause you to fall back into your binge eating or food addiction.

THE SOCIAL – It's important for you to have the family support you need to help you through this. Research shows when there are external supports in place the odds of success long-term improve immensely. Family counselling sessions will help you get better faster. This improves the communication between family aids in opening the mind and creating a more loving and sup-portive family unit.

Treatment Option Two - Meds
There is only one medication approved in the US specifi-cally geared towards the treatment of bulimia. Prozac or fluoxetine is also used for depression. It is quite common and chances are you've heard of it. Medical professionals report some patients with bulimia benefit with this drug treatment.

Treatment Option Three – Hospitalization
Understand, this is rare and extreme. But, if doctors feel there's a risk of suicide or self-harm, this is a viable op-tion.

Bulimia nervosa is a debilitating eating disorder that's of-ten difficult to diagnose and treat, simply because it isn't easily recognizable and most can hide it quite easily. Un-til the individual suffering comes forward and more importantly is ready and willing to seek treatment, there really isn't anything that can be done.

Often a loved one will recognize the symptoms and pose questions, only to be rejected and this accusation often triggers more denial and the walls around the suspected individual with bulimia solidify, so much so they will run further away from the truth at all cost.

Understand please the "accused" is scared, embarrassed, ashamed, humiliated and feels like a failure. You, of course, are trying to help and they are feeling vulnerable and attacked. This is how their mind is twisting things. So, be careful how you approach this issue if you suspect someone you care and love is suffering. Just so you know...

Anorexia Nervosa
This is a very serious and often life threatening food disorder, a mental disease where a dangerous low amount of food is eaten or a food aversion is present. This person often has seriously distorted perceptions of what they look like and actually develops a few so deep they believe eating anything is going make them fat. With their state of mind this is terrifying.

They become driven to lose weight no matter what, even if they are 5' and weigh just 80 pounds. It's the distorted belief of healthy weight and eating habits that fuel this health-robbing disease, a serious mental illness where appetite is lost or ignored that needs to be diagnosed and treated professionally. It most often strikes young teenagers and adults.

Suicide risk runs high and health experts from Stanford University Medical School report 1 in 10 sufferers die. *Why?*
It's a tough question to put a finger on. Most health specialists in the field believe the causal factors are mental, environmental and biological. Some may have personalities or genetic traits increasing the risk.

For example, if you are underweight and have "weird" eating habits, this could trigger your brain chemicals to program you for anorexia nervosa.

A few risk factors intertwined with anorexia:

Depression or anxiety
Extreme sensitivity to body image and weight
Bullied and teased about weight
Unsupportive environment in general
Family history
Overcautious and worried
Experienced any sort of eating issue
Societal pressures
Career in the limelight – celebrity
Perfectionist
Highly competitive gymnastics or cheerleading

Of course, the causal factors of anorexia nervosa aren't completely understood, what is known is that because of the gynormously controlling psychological component. Over time, this food addiction eating disorder becomes increasingly difficult to understand and treat. Quick intervention is your best move, aside from prevention and avoidance.

Signs and Symptoms
Someone suffering from anorexia is pressured to continuously hide their eating patterns. Often those affected, will wave off concerns for their health, but making up excuses that initially fools just about everyone. It's self-satisfaction for the time being. In time, the seriousness of this person's eating habits and severe weight loss will move to center stage. At this point, the scenario is entering the "deep" zone and action needs to be taken pronto.

FIRST

It's important to open your mind to recognizing these peculiar habits, whether with yourself, or a loved one. If you don't realize what is or might be going on here, then you can't get the help or offer the help required to develop a healthy relationship with food.

We're on the same page right?
If you find the scale number becomes a focal point, you start worrying about every single gram of fat you eat or start feeling negative about the way you look in the mirror, these need to be red flags in your mind along with…

Behavior Changes
Trying to lose weight when you're already a toothpick – Keep in mind this is subjective. Many women in particular judge another woman to be "too skinny" simply because they are unhappy with the rolls they are carrying around. There's no sugar coating that one. Perhaps I'll write a book about it one day!

But seriously, if you know you're thin enough and are still trying to lose weight or notice someone you realistically think is, then it's worth your while to address it.

Thoughts of "food" interfere with your daily routine – If you are happily trying to get your work done while ignoring your screaming tummy, with the continuous thoughts of "food" in your head, you've another red flag that could point to anorexia.

Set aside time to try and eat less food than you already are – If you already know the little food going to your body isn't sufficient and you are still trying to eat less, then you've a definitive symptom of anorexia.

Lying to yourself and others – If you find yourself repeatedly telling your friends at lunch you've already eaten when you haven't, or deny your hunger pains and explain you're full when your best friend offers to buy you lunch. You've stumbled upon, yet another symptom of this food addiction disorder.

Extreme change in habit – Changes in life that stick are gradual and continuous. A signal here might be when someone suddenly decides to not bother with your usually Friday night's out at the bar. Perhaps they decline every single social invitation with food.

Weirdo Behaviors – If your gut tells you someone is being weird, go with it. This could be anything from chewing food ten zillion times, setting the food on the plate a specific way or just getting organized to eat the EXACT same way every single time.

Image Changes
Extreme weight loss – There's cause for concern when anybody suddenly drops a whole whack of weight. It may be they've taken to eating healthy, exercising and taking care of themselves, sometimes though it's because they are in trouble and need help.

Feel fat and ugly no matter what – This is a tough feeling to accept. It's frustrating and doesn't make sense. But if you've feeling "fat," and you are quite the opposite, it's important you seek professional help. There's nothing good with a distorted body image regardless of the reason.

Your body weight and size consumes your every waking hour – If you find you just can't get the thoughts of how you look out of your head it's important you first recognize this isn't healthy. It's no wonder with the societal external pressures to be skinny these days, that girls in particular get focused to the extreme on how they look.

34

What's important is loving your body as it, flaws in all. Understanding no matter how much weight you lose their will AWAYS be something you aren't happy with. That's a fact!

Extremely critical of your body – You're only human right? If you find you are extra hard on being you, how you look and feel, then you need to pull into your conscious that you might be developing a mental disorder that needs professional attention, nothing to be embarrassed or ashamed about, rather you should be proud you've got the nerve to admit it and deal with it head on!

Sneakily convincing yourself you aren't extremely thin – This is really tough because it means you're going to have to admit you made a mistake and are wrong. Nobody likes to do that. When you are underweight by choice and won't admit it, then you've just solidified the fact you do need professional help. Get over it and get the help you need. Open your mind to the idea so you can get healthy and happy. It's exactly what you deserve!

Consequences
Anorexia nervosa has dire consequences on you physically and mentally. If you've body isn't getting the vital nutrients, vitamins and minerals it requires to function optimally, they will be health consequences over time. It's not just about having zero energy because your system has no complex carbs, lean protein or fat to break down for immediate energy. It's so much more than that.

A few of the consequences physically are:
*Nasty mood swings
*Depression
*Skin and hair issues, teeth and gum problems
*Issues with concentration and memory
*Weak nails

*Bowel issues
*"Downy" hair growing all over your body – just like a bear
*Lightheadedness and fainting
*Queasiness and vomiting
*Zilch in the energy level department
*Uncontrollable shaking

Anorexia affects you head to toe. With negative effects with your…
Hair
Brain
Nerves
Blood
Skin
Teeth
Hormones
Fluids
Kidneys
Joints and tendons
Muscles
Heart function
Intestines

As you can clearly see, anorexia nervous can't be ignored. You MUST take action!

Solutions/Treatment
Keep in mind here this food addiction disease is not like breaking your leg. In time your leg is mended and in most cases you're good to go and don't have to worry very much about breaking it again.

With anorexia there's a psychological component with technically means you will always have to be wary of your triggers long after you've beat it. Prevention is critical and this comes with understanding the signs and symptoms and ensuring proper treatment is executed. It won't be easy, but when you're sitting on the other side of the fence I can guarantee you'll be glad you had the courage to do it here, strategies to beat this disease once and for all!

Recognize and admit you have a problem and need help – This is the tough point, admitting to yourself and everyone else that you've taken a good intention to the extreme. Most of us could stand to lose a few pounds. When you take this to the extreme that it's unhealthy and damaging, that's when you need to admit this and stop.

Start openly talking about it – This step is gynormous. You'll feel a whole lot better about things after you finally openly admit your worries to a close friend or family member. You'll see you are welcome with open minds, understood and supported, with the focus of getting you well and soon as possible. Trust me on this one please.

Understand your triggers and avoid them – Changing your routine is a fabulous way to keep the triggers of anorexia away. Don't buy those pressurized-to-be-thin magazines or sit in on modelling shoots is that makes you focus on being thinner. The idea here is to set yourself up for success and if avoiding triggers helps you not think about the skinny thing, then do it!

Get professional help to create your plan – Probably the hardest factor here is actually admitting you need help. This isn't something you can beat on your own. Professional counselling will help you get to the root of the problem and create a successful plan that will set you up on the mend, the sooner the better here. Ignoring it will NOT make it go away.

Your mind, body and soul need to be addressed when battling anorexia. With the three focus steps being…

FINDING YOUR HEALTHY WEIGHT
SLOWLY EATING MORE HEALTHY FOODS
TRANFORMING SELF-THOUGHTS POSITIVE

Treatment Options…
Eating Advice – A nutritional counsellor will help you understand what nutrients your body needs, in what amounts and why. This is going to give you the "logic" behind eating more.

Counselling – This is a must to beat this psychological disease, understanding where your negative thoughts towards self-image and food come from is going to help you heal, creating a positive relationship with both food and your body, helping you to find the balance you need to thrive in health.

Medical Intervention – If you happen to be severely malnourished, dehydrated and stressed, medical inter-vention may be required. The purpose here is to stop weight loss and flip you both mentally and physically onto the weight gaining path. It's a must, if you want to live.

VIP Note – With anorexia nervosa, getting past the chal-lenge of even thinking about gaining weight (grotesque fat) is tough. Putting weight on is even tougher, simply because your head is still in the "must lose weight" frame of mind. So gaining weight even though you know you physically need to, is cause to feel like a failure.

This is a seriously deadly cycle of self-destruction that can be stopped. You are running the show here. First steps first. ADMIT you need help, they you can go about taking action and getting exactly what you need to put a smile no your face inside and out.

My Thoughts…
Bulimia and anorexia are more common than you think. This disease is sneaky difficult because it's both physical and mental. The mind is powerful and has the ability to be very sneaky. Society shuns eating disorders for the most part making it incredibly difficult to admit you are suffering one and get the professional help you need.

What you need to know is the general population sees things this way for the most part because they don't have the knowledge required to understand and relate to eat. These food addition disorders are not just found in the elite group of the rich and famous. They are NOT controllable when in full bloom, and those suffering aren't all rich and prissy, focused on being thin at all costs just because that's who they are.

That's all bull crap. ANYBODY can suffer from bulimia and anorexia. Truth be told, they're usually intertwined to some degree.

Boys and girls have it. Although it's primarily in young adolescent girls and young adults, that's not exclusive. Heck, grandma's and grandpa's might be suffering, moms and dads, sisters and brothers, aunts, uncles, friends and neighbors. Even children have been reported suffering.

It's time to open your mind and eyes. Take on the responsibility to become aware and take action if you are suffering. A choice you have to make…

Negative Effects of Food Addiction

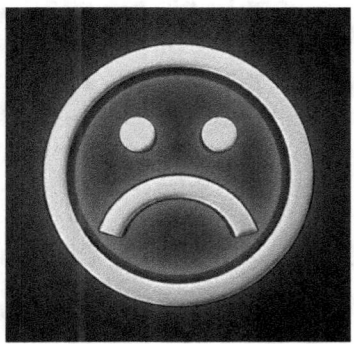

A food addiction is serious stuff, working to re-wire the same part of the brain affected by drug and alcohol abuse. It's all highly addictive and dangerous!

This Destructive Cycle Detailed...
Overdosing repeatedly on all the wrong foods doesn't just lead to unhealthy weight gain. It's like pulling the trigger to a domino effect game. Overtime eating the excessive Twinkies make you fat, steering you away from the gym because you lack confidence in you, embarrassed by your body image. These negative discouraging thoughts lead further to depression. And you look to adding tubs of ice cream to your daily routine to help soothe your blues away. Fat, feeling lethargic and ugly you now refrain from socializing with your friends, so disappointed in yourself you flip these self-loathing thoughts around and assume your friends wouldn't want to hang out with you because you're not perfect.

The pure thought of this is most unbearable, forcing you deeper into the endless cycle of eating, guilt, regret, sadness, shame and blame. You decide to start binging to temporarily rid yourself of your physically bursting and very uncomfortable sugar loaded gut, along with mentally clearing your conscience because you've undone the damage "in the moment." This may be enough to even go out with friends before you whole yourself up in secrecy for another round, feeling temporarily "okay" because you've figured out a way to "have your cake and eat it too" without the consequence of getting fatter. Of course you don't give a rat's ass right now about any other consequences of binge eating. You turn your head to them and continue on. Figuring soon you'll just stop, but it never happens.

Food addiction negatively affects you mentally, physically, socially and emotionally, interfering with not only you every day, but also all that you could be if you were healthy.

That's the longer version of the viscous cycle of emotionally charged food addiction.

Mental/Emotional Negatives
*Increased psychological stress
*Feeling of failure
*Lack of self-confidence
*Depression
*Anxiety issues
*Roller-coaster moods
*No belief to achieve dreams
*Poor work/school performance
*"Happiness" only interconnected with sugary high-fat foods in gynormous quantities or regularly/patterned
*Unhealthy stress – self-created
*Lying patterns develop and manifest

42

*Fear of food and eating too much at any given time – the wrong time when others are around

Physical Negatives
*Gaining weight
*Increase risk cardiovascular disease, stroke and diabetes
*High blood pressures and cholesterol
*Greater chance of developing kidney disease, bone issues, sleep issues and arthritis

Social Negatives
*Isolation (to eat in privacy)
*Relationship issues
*Loss of interest in hobbies (eating instead)
*Becomes uncomfortable in social "food" situations for fear of spilling the beans
*Fear of close interaction with others – increases chances of someone finding out

My Thoughts…
The physical, mental, emotional and social consequences associated with emotional eating or food addiction are very real. Unfortunately, each negative is interconnected with the other, creating a chain of devastation, not just one isolated event.
What's important to recognize is that you can put a stop to it. Mind over matter works but it will take time, a plan, support and professional guidance. And most importantly you've got to WANT to send you food addiction packing. YOU have to choose that, nobody else.

Tips to Avoid – Stop Food Addiction BEFORE It Manifests Into Reality

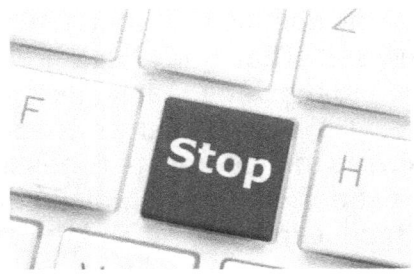

Even though the media sends the message loud and clear that negative relationships with food equates eventually into serious health issues, we still continue full steam ahead, teasing our palates with high fat sweets, greasy fast food and other nutrition-less processed foods that just weigh us down. We teach our taste buds to crave unnatural sugary foods in lieu of the nutrients, vitamins and minerals required for optimal health.

STOP and think about these pointers before food addiction moves in for good.

Define clearly wants/needs/desires. It's not good enough just to say you to lose weight and get healthy. That just doesn't cut it, because you're too vague and uncommitted.

Stop and really think about what you want? Why you want to stop or keep yourself from spiraling out of control with unhealthy foods. Maybe you want to stop avoiding

45

your friends? Gain control of your moods? Find untapped energy?

Point is you need to be realistic and sincere if you want to create a positive relationship with food and keep it that way.

Don't break what isn't broke. You don't need to reinvent the wheel here. Pay attention to what naturally slim people do and follow suit. They don't have "forbidden" foods, a disaster waiting to happen for any black sheep out there. They will eat some unhealthy sweets from time to time, but just always in moderation. A healthy "learned" habit for life. No stress, no thought. Make the time to feel and taste your food, experience it and the appreciation will come.

Respect what *you want.* If you have cravings DO NOT ignore them. This is about being true to you. Honest with yourself. If you *really* want to eat something, don't blindly deny yourself.

Condition yourself to want less over time. It's about learning a new "normal" for you. So if you want to get rid of your craving for deep delicious melt in your mouth triple chocolate fudge double layer cake you've become accustomed to every night after your late night munchies. Then it's logical to say if you just stopped cold turkey, it's highly likely you're not going to make it stick. Why? Your expectations are commendable but not realistic.

Humans are creatures of habit. This means you're intrinsically programmed to resist change. We love routine and creating new habits isn't easy.

To do this you've got to warm your way into your new expectation. With the delicious cake, try having it every other night to start, respecting your "old" ways of eating while introducing your new healthier intentions.

This allows your "psychological" to be content and your physiological addiction to this sugary tweet to be satisfied but sent in a healthier direction. In time you'll reduce this addiction even more. Simultaneously you can substitute something healthier if you like. Perhaps some fresh fruit with a dalop of whipped topping to start, or if you really want something sweet, a few caramel rice cakes or graham crackers with a smear of peanut butter.

The sky is the limit here. Just ensure that you don't deny yourself completely, particularly right off the top. This will backfire and likely only escalate your particular food addiction. You don't have to deny yourself, just be strong in moderation, your limits and in creative ingenuity.

Learn to recognize and better control your emotions. Experts agree across the board it's those pesky emotions that often trigger food addictions or what may refer to as "emotional eating."

Chances are good you've experienced this personally, just maybe not to the degree of it transforming into a mental condition. Perhaps when your girlfriend dumped you, feelings of sadness overwhelmed, directing you to drown your sorrows in tubs of your favorite chocolate ice cream while watching your favorite chick-flics for a week straight? When you lost your job you may have tried to pretend it didn't matter that you know have no way to pay your bills. So you decided just for the fun of it to go on a major drinking and "junky eating" food binge for a week to cope.

Both of these instances are prime examples of emotional eating, where your emotions area raging out of control and you turn to food to try and regain it, which of course doesn't work. If you don't recognize this and learn to control it, there's a good chance it will become habit and more likely to happen, something that only escalates with time.

Once this coping mechanism is established it's incredibly hard to remove. Stopping it before it starts is your best move.

 Here are a few indicators suggesting you're in the danger zone of emotional eating.

*You eat without thinking, even when your tummy's not rumbling.

*Your eating is automated, like when you're watching a movie you ALWAYS gobble down an extra-large double butter popcorn with a cherry coke soda.

*It's obvious certain emotions lead you to the refrigerator, pantry or closest fast-food drive-thru.

*It's hard for you to "feel" satisfied when eating. This means your mind and body are out of sync, enabling you to eat and eat and still not be satisfied.

*You are emotionally volatile. With the flick of a switch, you can be out of control emotionally. At this point, it's too late as you're already knee deep in the junk food.

Newsflash!
There's a very important biological component that ties food to our emotions. It's one many people aren't aware of. It really is quite simple. When stressed, your internal systems are saturated in the hormone cortisol, which is a known trigger for high sugar car-

48

bohydrates, unhealthy carbs that shoot your blood sugar levels through the roof, along with your logic. Eating immediately changes the chemical balance of your body, soothing your emotions and giving you a VERY short-lived "feel good" feeling, like an endorphin release. That happens when you exercise with intensity. Just think "runners high" here.

It's that same "addictive" feeling, except you quickly come crashing down to earth and feel like a dirty bag of bricks.

It's also imperative you recognize eating for other reason than actually being physically hungry, all of which can be the seeds of food addiction, something you want to steer clear of if at all possible.

Some more are...
*Boredom – If you're simply eating because you've got nothing better to do, please stop it! Find a hobby, hang out with friends or go clean your house. Fill your time with anything other than eating.

*Learned "Feel Good"- You may have been taught to feel all warm and cozy inside eating your mom's homemade fudge cake, or maybe you used to make fantabulous deep fried chicken balls in butter, associated unhealthy foods with positive feelings is a ticking time bomb waiting to explode if you let it get out of hand.

*Social Pressures – Here, you might work with people that eat fried foods every lunch and line up at the vending machine every break. Be aware it doesn't take long to reach "food addiction" state and then you're in trouble.

*Learned Beliefs – Right or wrong doesn't matter with this one. What you believe is what you believe. Perhaps

you're obsessed with Beyonce, and she happens to en-
dorse McDonald's Big Mac and fries. If you eat that every
day because you are so hooked with that gorgeous girl,
then you've allowed your beliefs in someone you don't
even "know," steer you down the path towards unhealthy
food addiction, that'll likely also turn you into a "tubby."
It's something Beyonce is definitely not. Makes you wonder, doesn't it?

My Thoughts…
Food addiction is something you don't want to get into,
when emotion and logic tango it's tough to come out on
top. By recognizing "how" food addiction begins, you'll
better arm yourself with the mind-power required to side-
step carefully here, ensuring you never do too much of
any one episode of unhealthy eating. This ensures the
red flags are in place to keep you from stepping over the
edge to the point of "extremely difficult" return.

Solutions to Food Addiction

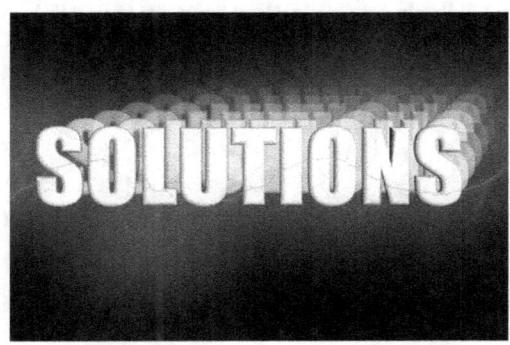

Food addiction hurts. It's controlling. It can make you physically it, and eventually can lead to your early demise.

Food addiction triggers emotional craziness, extreme changes in your moods due to blood sugar instability and psychological stresses. This addiction manifests over time, escalating to the point in which it dictates your every move.

Each of these facts is hurtful, and when you are physically and mentally ready to beat it. Here is a plan, the *mindset* tools you need to take action and win!

Self-medicating with food is extremely dangerous and highly addictive, based on the fact simple sugars are crazy-nuts addictive. When we choose foods to go overboard on to ineffectively "cure" troublesome life challenges, we go for the goods. Sweet bakery items, chips, soda, candy bars and pounds of fast food fat seem to be the nourishment of choice without thought. Of course, our mind is temporarily happy because it's always a challenge to play the "black sheep" of the family for a while, right?

It's no secret these foods are in no way, shape or form "good" for us. They spike blood sugars temporarily, instigate moods swings and uncontrollable emotions, because depression, increasing anxiety, trigger disease and force our body to run on "crappy" fuel. In time, this will kill us. We know all this, but there just seems to be something internally and unconsciously programmed into us to "want that bad boy."

Well the "bad boy," or girl is sugar, which would be fine if it was once in a while and in moderation. Probably, it isn't. In the blink of an eye, this exciting experimentation on the dark side will grab hold of you and handcuff you, forcing a battle of wills within.

What makes it difficult is the fact we LOVE the temporary "feeling fabulous" feeling we get with all this crap-loaded junk food in our system. THAT is the addiction that keeps us coming back.

THE TRUTH?
If we want something bad enough in life, we WILL cleverly find a way to get it. You know, it, I know it and hopefully soon the whole world will.

Overeating or food addiction is a disease. If you want to control and manage it you need to set out a serious game plan and implement. Going through the motions will just fuel the fire here. Trust me on this on. Been there ~ done that!

Useful Steps/Stages to Break the Viscously Nasty Cycle of Food Addiction

Consciously Program Change

There's no ifs, ands or buts about it. Humans are creatures of habit and we find welcome comfort in routine, regardless of just what that is. Think about it for a minute. Content infants thrive in a routine that works like clockwork. There's so much in their sweet and precious life they do have control over. That knowing when they're going to eat and nap and get their bum changed is comforting to them. Sure it changes, but with their cue as they grow and their needs change.

Children are the best with a routine. There's no doubt about it. Mine are living, breathing proof. Many of my friends have children that aren't!

So routine serves a purpose in a positive sense, but also stands as a barrier when it's important you take the initiate to make a change. Does that make sense?
We are naturally resistant to change and this is something that needs to be recognized, teleported from unconsciousness to consciousness and engaged. You need to stand up to your resistance and TELL yourself you need to change. Convince yourself first before anything else. It's the mental here you need to take charge of. Be a bully for a moment in time for all the right reasons.

Your health is important and this means YOU need to trigger change, or your cycle will never be broken. Sad, but true.

Positive Affirmation is a fabulous tool here, where you will repeatedly tell yourself, morning noon and night, that positive things are going to happen when you make changes. Remind yourself you are strong, beautiful, successful, courageous and you need to make these changes to get yourself healthy and capable of so much more in life.

Write these positive affirmations on your mirror in red hot lipstick, post-it notes on your desk, in a journal and maybe even on your refrigerator door. Point is you need to commit to the first step here which is re-programming yourself here, brain first, to open your mind to change and actually accept it without a fight.

REALITY – Is this going to be challenging?
Absolutely.
Is it doable?
That's another affirmative!
It's up to you to make the first move. You are in control and you get to choose.

Flip YOUR Switch to Positive
There's no doubt here that you will give yourself some grief here, looking for reasons NOT to change, trying to tell yourself it was just so much easier drowning your sorrows in chocolate covered strawberries and gallons of triple chocolate marsh mellow ice cream with hot fudge and a handful of cherries.

DON'T let yourself get sucked in. Tell yourself you know the feeling of happiness eating all that is only temporary. Shortly after you will feel like a piece of shit and deep in that loathsome barrel of crap than you were before. Keep telling yourself you don't want to re-live all those negative feelings associated with food addiction. It's just not worth it.

EXPECT you are going to challenge yourself here and be ready for it. Flip each of these sabotaging thoughts to positive and soar. Fly to the top of the highest velvety

54

cloud close to the beautiful sunshine and get a refreshing sun-kissed tan.

Don't stop and ensure your mind won't accept any sort of deviant behavior that's going to send you back to square one. Set your mind on positive and commit to making it work and then some.

Realize Your Triggers
Unless you connect the dots here and consciously recognize your triggers to overeating, you're pretty much sunk in the deepest part of the deep blue sea. Most eat for emotional reasons. Figure yours out and be ready. Identify them and write them down, forcing yourself to make the association between sadness and creampuffs or corn chips and frustration. Do you see what I'm getting at here?

Recognizing your triggers is going to give you the knowledge to advance in the battle and take action. You are courageous enough, aren't you?

Stand Strong – It Gets Easier
This is a tough one, but it's important to have the mindset you are strong and can "wait" out the storm. Of course, the "storm" being those irresistible urges to stick your face in a chocolate fountain when depressed, or to fill yourself so full of fast foods that you nearly explode every Friday night after work religiously.

Just grin and bear it, not participating of course. It won't take you long to realize the uncontrollable urges will subside if you just allow them to take their course.
Understand you've create an expectation for your body to get overdosed with sugars on specific occasions. It didn't just come up with this craving on its own. You communicated and provided and now you've got to re-teach

yourself NOT to expect the triple fudge chocolate sundae every afternoon after your two hour siesta.

EXPECT there will some unpleasantries before you start feeling good again. This prepares your mind to just deal with it, understanding it does get better.

Cut the Power Source
Here, you must commit to cutting off all sources of power in empowering your food addiction. This means when one of your "oh-so-powerful" negative emotions pop into the picture. You DO NOT fuel it with sugar or other fatty foods in the extreme.

It's important you make no exceptions to the rule here or you are just going to reaffirm to your body, mind and confidence that you are a big fat failure and might as well just live in sugary misery forever.

NOT TRUE!
With a little patience and a whole lot of perseverance, you WILL slowly drain the power from your cravings, finding they are less overwhelming and easier to control. *Newsflash* – Did you know that by eating a sweet snack when you're hungry, tying yourself over till dinner, TEACHES your body to crave sugar before healthy foods? So instead of grabbing a candy bar while dinners cooking or a slice of chocolate cake, you should opt for a plate of veggies, slice of whole grain bread with peanut butter or maybe a handful of nuts, that way you're not fueling the fire, brewing up more trouble in the food addiction dilemma.

Focus Switch
One of the most successful ways to remove a negative behavior is by not focusing on it. Instead, start replacing it

and essentially pushing it out of your life by filling your plate up with positive ones.

Over time, these positive repeated actions will turn habit and you just won't have room for the negative ones and out the window they'll go without a parachute.
So let's say you normally hit the vending machine with your bosom buddies every lunch hour, of course excited to see what sugary sweets on the menu to help muck up your internal circuits.

Why not slip in with the lunch walkers and spend your lunch hour walking the city instead of basking in the short-lived glow of a dangerous sugar high? Pack your lunch and eat it while you walk, ALL healthy, of course. This way you are eating lean protein, healthy carbs and essential vitamins and minerals your body requires AND you are expending more energy by walking. It's a double win for you and trust me on this one. You're soon going to feel and look like ten million bucks!

No Excuses
Many have a hard time succeeding with beating their food addiction simply because they CHOOSE not to get rid of their professional degree in excuse making. Excuses are the easy route and you get NOTHING accomplished using them.

Yes, we're all guilty.
Recognize you are human and have learned to make excuses when you don't want to bother dealing with a situation and/or your feelings.

Set your mind to expect there are going to be obstacles thrown in your path and instead of making excuses, consciously CHOOSE to just find the solution.

For example: The social always seems to get us into trouble with eating. If you haven't seen your good friend for a while now and KNOW you're both going to end up in the ice cream shop over-indulging. DO NOT use the fact you haven't seen her for a while as an excuse to feed your food addiction.

Supports
Don't think for one minute you need to tackle your emotional eating or food addiction on your own. Having supports in place is what you need to succeed. BELIEVE IT!

Professional counselling is important to help create a strategy to re-gig your brain to not want extreme amounts of sugar. To help remove the thoughts that support your out of control eating. Psychological counselling has the expertise in helping with this.

Having family and friends on board is also important. Your environment can interfere with or support progress. A supportive, loving and understanding environment will help you hold to your goals. You'll be less likely to fall backwards and more likely to dig deep to get control of your food addiction.

This reminds you that you aren't alone, very important when challenging the unknown and looking for your new way.

My Thoughts…
You and I both know change isn't easy. Understanding there are solid steps you must take in order to beat your food addiction is critical. Knowing what to expect is half the battle. It's when you are blindsided that usually hurts.

Using these strategies and steps to help build the mind confidence to switch your negative learned eating habits to positive, is all good.
Teach your mind to always flip even the most difficult scenarios to positive and soon you WILL believe you can create your reality. Hard, but doable. You've got to stick to it!

Final Thoughts

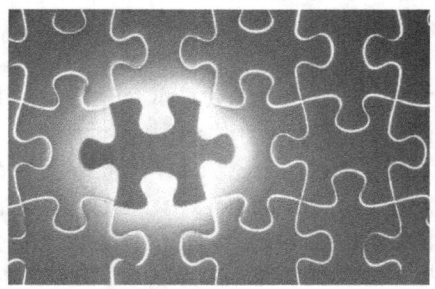

Nobody wants to admit they have a food addiction. In fact, nobody really wants to admit anything another might deem as "negative" or "weak." That's just natural. But the fact is we all have weakness and it's safe to say most of us have this with food.

It doesn't mean we all have a food addiction, but because we can't live without food it's important we are each aware of the triggers and solutions to this worldwide epidemic. This way we can use preventative measures and/or have the tools necessary to get a handle on our food addiction to stop it from interfering with and eventually gaining control of our life. I'm sure you can relate.

Recognize that stress and emotion often get out of hand in the world today, both of which trigger emotional eating, instead of listening to our body and eating when we truly are hungry. We start teaching our body to use food as an emotional condolence, to help soothe anxiety and stress, temporarily diffuse sadness and substitute for a shoulder to cry on, when all we really need is just that.

We're on dangerous ground when we look to food for anything other than providing optimal fuel for our body and mind to function, eating "bad" or high-fat sugary fuel, or rather teaching our mind and body to crave it, will only interfere with our good health, physically, mentally, emotionally and socially.

It's ironic we consciously know all this, but allow it to happen anyway. Just doesn't make sense.
What's important here is that you understand the dangers of food addiction and have the tools to beat it. The choice is yours, if you want to take control of your eating and not let it negatively control you. Now you have the tools at your fingertips to do just that. Time for you to get to it, don't you think?

You know you can and you've got the "know-how." Now it's just a matter of whether you've got the "will" to or no. My opinion is you most certainly do! It's your call.

In order for my books to rank and sell on Amazon they need positive reviews. If you enjoyed my book and have a few minutes to write a 3-5 line review about my book, that would really help me. Thank you :)

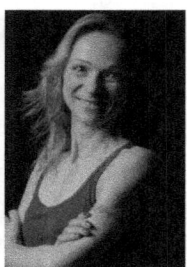

I hope that you enjoyed my book and you can check out all my other books by visiting my website at: flawlesscreativewriting.com

Disclaimer

www.ingramcontent.com/pod-product-compliance
Lightning Source LLC
Chambersburg PA
CBHW070323290526
45791CB00003B/1235